Disclaimer

This e-book has been written to provide information about self-improvement.

Every effort has been made to make this eBook as complete and accurate as possible. However, there may be mistakes in typography or content.

Also, this e-book provides information only up to the publishing date. Therefore, this eBook should be used as a guide - not as the ultimate source.

The purpose of this eBook is to educate.

The author and the publisher do not warrant that the information contained in this e-book is fully complete and shall not be responsible for any errors or omissions.

The author and publisher shall have neither liability nor responsibility to any person or entity with respect to any loss or damage caused or alleged to be caused directly or indirectly by this e-book.

About the Author

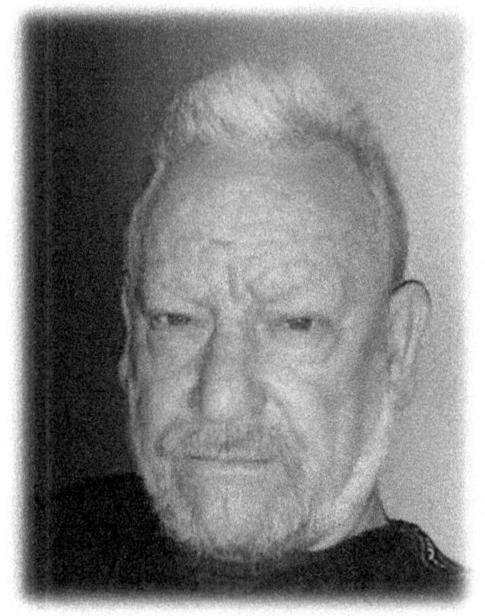

Simon Sézé is an accomplished business executive who has worked for several major corporations and has started his own businesses. He is a self-improvement guru who believes that anything is possible with clarity of intent and strength of purpose.

Working with his clients to uncover their true potential, he emphasizes self-honesty and constant balance, steering away from the burnout and exhaustion that are so common among highly motivated people.

Simon Sézé has seen time and again what happens when people are willing to fight for their visions. He strives to impact the world in a positive way and to effect mindset shifts that lead to greater productivity and lower energy expenditure simultaneously.

Introduction

Anyone can come up with a goal, but not everyone has the ability to achieve it. For that to happen, you need to take action first. Goals are not like dreams or prayers. You cannot just close your eyes and wish for it to happen. You have to do something.

But of course, it does not end there. Certainly, taking the first step toward reaching your goal is the most crucial but it is not the only thing you have to do. There are a lot more steps to take and you have to work hard, and for that you need to be focused.

You need to learn how to ignore distraction. Perhaps in a perfect world, no person would have to be subjected to distraction when trying to accomplish a goal. But this is reality, and distraction comes in all shapes and sizes.

Sometimes, distraction comes from within. This is the insidious of distractions because how do you ignore something that lives inside your mind or heart? This is when motivation kicks in. As the old adage goes, *when the going gets tough, the going gets tougher.*

• Goals are like a destination that you have to reach.

• Taking action is what gives you direction toward your goal.

• Staying focused ensures that you are always on the right path.

• And lastly, motivation is what makes sure that you will do anything and everything to reach the end of the path, arrive at your destination, and achieve your goal.

This is a never ending and rather flexible cycle. At times, you will need to motivate yourself in order to take action. Other times, you need to take action to stay focused. Which goes first does not matter so do not be surprised if you find yourself jumping from one tip to another.

What matters is that you are taking all the positive steps toward reaching your goal. So, if you are ready to finally make your goal come true, then here goes!

Tips for Taking Action

Tip 1: Just do it

The first step is always the hardest. Your mind will come up with all sorts of scenarios to prevent you from taking that scary first step toward your goal. That does not mean you are a coward, though. It is just your brain's way of defending yourself.

Sometimes you have to listen to what your heart has to say and just do it. Everything else will be a lot easier once you get past the first hurdle – and that is to ignore your brain's dire warnings and go with your gut instinct.

Tip 2: Doing something is not always a physical action

Don't confuse the need for taking action as doing something literally or physically. There are many other ways for you to take action without ever lifting a finger. For instance, consider the act of planning.

It is never wise to try achieving a goal without a plan. If you want to spend the least amount of time and effort in achieving your goal, then you need to come up with a step-by-step plan for accomplishing it.

A good plan takes into account all potential consequences as well as all the possible avenues you may take in order to reach your objective.

Tip 3: Breathing helps

Are you feeling nervous or nauseous? Does the effort to reach your goal stress you out? It is normal to feel uneasy about tackling a challenging goal. Taking action is often synonymous to taking risk. You are nervous because you know that risks can either end with success or failure, and who wants to end up failing?

Whenever you feel like there is a panic attack coming on, just take a deep breath. Better yet, take several deep breaths. Studies show how breathing can effectively clear the mind and help calm your nerves. Go ahead and breathe - inhale all the way from your stomach to take full advantage!

Tip 4: Take a page from the most successful books

You may think that you are the only one suffering a certain kind of problem, but you are not. With a little research, you are sure to find something in common with ordinary and extraordinary people.

Look around you. If you are authentic and open about your challenges you are bound to find someone in a similar situation.

Tip 5: Take baby steps

Be your own person. Do not push yourself to achieve the same things others have done in the same way they did. In the end, you have to remind yourself that every person is unique and, consequently, has their own set of strengths and weaknesses.

Also, it could be that you are just starting out and the other person you are comparing yourself to is years ahead of you in terms of expertise and experience. The other person cannot afford to take baby steps, but you can, and you should!

If you rush things too much, everything may end up backfiring on you.

Tip 6: Rome wasn't built in a day

This is obviously related to the previous tip, but it is different in the way that it takes into account what you want to do with your time.

It is good to have a plan for everything, but you do not have to accomplish everything in a single day. Even if you have the energy to do so, those around you (family members, co-workers) who have a stake in reaching your shared goals may not have the time and similar energy to do so.

Give them a break. If all of you work hard, then you all deserve to rest. There is always tomorrow.

Tip 7: Do not pressure yourself

Pressuring yourself is different from motivating yourself. Motivating yourself will get you to take action while pressuring yourself will only succeed in paralyzing yourself.

There are going to be others in your life that will try to pressure you about getting things done. Why burden yourself with more pressure when you can give yourself a pep talk instead?

Tip 8: A little competition is good – just do not make a big deal out of it

Competition can motivate you because the more you delay, the further behind you will be in achieving your goal. Friendly competition is also effective for staying focused and getting you pumped up, but be careful!

If you let yourself focus too much on the competition, then you may end up forgetting about the bigger picture. In the end, being too

competitive may be another source of distraction
that you absolutely do not need.

Tip 9: Believe in yourself

Taking action requires you to have faith in
yourself – especially if people around you are
telling you that you cannot do it. Remember no
one know you better than yourself. You know
what you are capable of. If you believe that the
goal you have in mind is well within your reach,
then it truly is – no matter what others may say.

Tip 10: Get a companion

Just because you have someone with you and
willing to help you out doesn't imply that you are
not strong enough to accomplish your goal. It
also does not make your goal any less satisfying.
If anything, the goal becomes sweeter because
you have someone to share it with!

If you feel that you need your spouse or best
friend to be at your side to accomplish a
particular goal, then go and make it happen with
them.

Tip 11: Get someone to do it for you

Taking action also does not mean that you have
to do everything alone. Say your goal is to build a
house. Does that mean you should do

everything, from pouring concrete to installing shingles? Of course not!

Taking action may also mean finding the best person to do the job. Do not be shy about admitting that something is well beyond your actual KSAs (knowledge, skills, and abilities). There are just some things in life that are better left in the hands of an expert.

Tip 12: Do not be too proud to ask for help

A lot of people confuse taking action as doing something that directly
contributes to achieving a specific goal. What they fail to understand is that sometimes, indirect actions also matter just as much.

Sometimes that action is just an internal mental shift. For instance, the act of forgetting about your pride. Some people may say that it has nothing to do with achieving a goal, but what if it is your pride that is holding you back from getting much-needed help from an expert?

Tip 13: It is okay to start again

What if there comes a point in time that you realize that the first step you took was actually the wrong one? Or what if you suddenly realize that what you are doing is not taking you toward your goal but away from it?

If this happens, the only action you SHOULD NOT take is quitting.

If you realize that something is wrong, then clear your mind and retrace your steps until you find out what critical mistake you committed. Correct it and move on. If you have to, start from scratch – the sooner, the better!

Tip 14: Never stop trying!

As mentioned earlier on, the process of achieving one's goal is never ending. Taking action also means that you have to get back on your feet if you stumble. It is even okay if you have to start all over again. In the end, what is critical is that you do not let your failures keep you from continuously taking action and moving forward.

Pick yourself up, dust off, and learn from your mistakes. You will be a better and stronger person for doing this!

Tip 15: Have a back-up plan

Plans – just like rules – can be broken. And you need to be prepared for that eventuality right from the start by having a back-up plan ready.

Others feel that back-up plans are akin to admitting failure. It is not. Rather, back-up plans are actually a smart way of acknowledging the fact that change is the only thing that is constant in the world. There is no way for you to predict what is going to happen in the next minute, but you *can* try to prepare for things that could happen.

Tip 16: Consider your resources

Taking action gives you direction but that is not what it is all about. You also have to consider the resources you have on hand. How do you make the most out of them? What other resources do you need in order to make a move? Where can you get it?

Willpower and motivation, as well as focus, are all great things to have but these are *internal* resources. You also have to back up your plan with external and concrete resources like money, manpower, and skills.

Tip 17: Look before you leap but leap all the same!

There are two kinds of risks: manageable and unmanageable. You are lucky if all the steps in your action plan are manageable risks. What if they are not? Should you stop and let all your previous hard work go to waste?

Risks are scary, and it is a good thing that you are aware of them. Those who think they can take on any kind of risk are simply foolhardy and reckless. That is not courage, it is a lack of wisdom.

If you come across an unmanageable risk or a risk where the stakes are too high, do look before you leap. Consider the ups and downs, but most importantly of all – consider what your brain and guts have to say. Then leap – and leap high – if you really need to!

<u>Tip 18: Do not be too rigid or stubborn</u>

You have to know when to give up and change tactics. On paper, your plan may look fool proof and absolutely brilliant, but a lot of things in the real world are unpredictable and derail your plan.

You have to know when to stop knocking yourself against the wall and find another way toward reaching your goal. Remember: when there is a will, there is a way. If your Plan A did not work, what else is your Plan B good for if you are not willing to use it?

<u>Tip 19: Do not wait for things to happen. Make it happen instead!</u>

The most successful people I know are always active participants. Instead of passively waiting, hoping, and wishing that something would happen to them – they are proactive and make things happen.

They are not the kind to wait for a sign from the fates or a falling star to appear before they get moving. If they have a goal in sight, and they have a plan for achieving it, then they will move heaven and earth to get it.

<u>Tip 20: Give yourself a reasonable deadline</u>

Existing commitments may be a valid reason slowing the progress toward your goal. You also have to understand that some of these commitments are never going to go away. They

are there for life. Don not let these
"commitments" keep you from taking necessary
action.

You have to be firm with yourself and give
yourself a deadline. It may be a date further out
than you wanted. Sometimes, that is the only
way to get things done.

Tip 21: Be decisive

When you do commit yourself to a plan of action
be decisive about it. This keeps your progress
steady and make it easier for you to achieve your
goal. If you are in a leadership position, people
are unlikely to have faith in your decision if they
can see your faith and commitment wavering.

You have to show them that you know what
needs to be done and you have the power to
help everyone reach their goals – if they follow
you.

Tips for Staying Focused!

Tip 22: Make a checklist

Checklists show you where you are, how much you have progressed, and what still needs to be done in order to achieve your goal.

Even if you suddenly fall sick and have to leave the office for a week, the moment you get back your checklist will be enough to bring you up to speed.

Tip 23: Set a schedule

The quickest way to reaching your goal is to schedule your action steps – and stick to it. How many hours each day can you truly set aside for reaching your goal? What part of the day is the best time to work on reaching your goal?

A schedule also means having a specific place for you to do your work. Choose something that will benefit the kind of work that you are doing and the kind of person you are. Will something peaceful and quiet work more for you or do you prefer to be working outdoors and surrounded by sounds of nature?

Tip 24: Make it a habit

It is not enough, of course, to simply make a schedule. Creating one is easy – it is the "doing" part that is difficult. To easily stick to your schedule, you have to turn it into a habit. Treat it as an integral part of your day that you absolutely cannot miss.

Your body does not automatically search for caffeine in the morning just because it wants to. It was trained to do so by repetitive action, strengthened by your own desire for a delicious cup of coffee. Your mind also does not look for its daily fix of quiz shows in the evenings for no reason. It was trained to do so as well.

So why can't you train yourself to make your goal achievement schedule a part of your daily routine as well?

Tip 25: No excuses!

It is critical that you do not make any excuses. If you do, then the excuses will never stop. Your body has a "giving-in" muscle and every time you give in, it gets more powerful. Before you know it, that muscle has been flexed so much that it is impossible to ignore.

Tip 26: If you really have to, then it is okay to negotiate the terms – but do keep your word

There are times when no matter how hard you try, you just cannot find the energy to do the work. Or perhaps you are too occupied or excited by something else that your goal focus is pushed to the back of your mind.

At times like this, there really is no other option left but to "negotiate" the terms of your schedule. If you planned to work four hours today yet you can only work three, then work an extra hour tomorrow or the day after.

It is important to specify the date for your negotiated term and to keep your word to yourself. This, however, is one thing that you absolutely must not make into a habit!

Tip 27: Eliminate distraction.

Distraction is your focus' greatest enemy. Like temptation, it is insidious and will find all sorts of ways to mess with your concentration. Before you even start working, you should start by eliminating all possible sources of distraction.

Distraction can also be internal. These are those lingering doubts and worries that do nothing to help you reach your goal. Practice pushing them to the back of your mind. Keep practicing and they soon won't be a bother at all!

Tip 28: Log out from all social networking and social messaging systems

Maybe you find lots of great information and stay connected with your network or market by keeping yourself online. Surely your personal life or business can exist for a few hours without being glued to Twitter and Facebook.

No matter how you look at it, Twitter, Facebook, forums and all the other ways to communicate with people online will only be a potential source of distraction.

When you schedule says it is goal focus time, then focus!

Tip 29: Meditate

Numerous studies have already proven that meditation techniques – just like breathing exercises – are helpful in clearing your mind *and* improving your focus. If your emotions or pressures of the day is making it difficult for you to concentrate, meditating may get you re-focused.

You do not need to chant any mantras to meditate – although if you feel it will help, go ahead and do so. Just find a quiet place to sit and close your eyes and let your mind wander freely.

Do *not* lie down while meditating as you may end up sleeping instead. This tip comes from the voice of experience!

Tip 30: Take a time-out but limit it!

Sometimes, you can get burned out if you have been working too hard, too long. When this happens, it is okay to take a little breather from your schedule.

Time-outs cannot last forever. Make sure you time it to short break. If you are working only for a few hours, then ten to fifteen minutes should be enough. If, however, your schedule encompasses the whole day, then take an hour at most. Anything longer than that may drain your enthusiasm to get back to work.

Tip 31: Are You Sleeping Enough?

According to the experts, sleep can have a significant impact on your ability to concentrate. Having enough hours of sleep will improve your concentration. Having too little, or even too much of it, may create problems with staying focused.

To get enough sleep every night, you should try keeping regular hours or at least have a fixed schedule for sleep.

Tip 32: Diet matters

Diet also has a lot to do with your ability to stay focused. A healthy meal plan for the day will go a long way in improving your mind's ability to work and increase your stamina. Make sure you also take in enough vitamins and minerals as well. If necessary, take health supplements.

Tip 33: Exercise matters as well

You may think that exercising has nothing to do with helping you reach your goals but actually it does.

At least that is what most scientific studies are suggesting. Like meditating and sleeping, a sufficient amount of daily exercise will also help improve the state of your mind. That you will get fitter and look more fabulous are just icing on the cake!

Tip 34: Enjoy what you are doing.

Find a way to make the process of achieving your goal enjoyable. Sometimes it only takes a change of scenery. Other times, you just have to find the right perspective to look at your situation.

When you are doing something you love, such as cooking, reading, or dancing, or your favourite hobby, then you have no problems concentrating, right? But if you are being forced to do something you hate, it seems like anything can take your mind off your work.

Tip 35: How about a change of pace?

Focus is also dependent on pace. You may be trying to do things too fast or too slow for your brain to actually *enjoy* what you are doing.

When your pace is punishingly fast, you are more liable to commit mistakes. In your effort to save yourself time, you may be causing yourself to suffer greater delays since some of your tasks have to be redone or rectified.

Using an excessively slow or relaxing pace may not be the best answer either. Do not overestimate your ability to get some things done. Doing so might develop into procrastination.

Tip 36: Consider a change of setting

Sometimes, working in the same place day in and day out can get a little boring, and your mind will start to wander. When you have tried your best to stay focused and you just can't, then a change of setting may be in order.

Look for a different place – just for a day or two – to go when it is time to work on your goal. A new place may be enough to rekindle your interest. It may also help get your creativity flowing and give you an idea or two on how to better motivate yourself.

Tip 37: Be methodical

One of the best ways to stay focused is to be methodical. Do not choose a random point to start working toward your goal. Whatever it is you are aiming for – even if it is to improve your marriage or lose weight – there is sure to be a methodical or logical system for doing it.

Taking a methodical approach helps improve your focus because it enables you to see where you are going. If you are feeling a little stuck or not sure of what to do next, a just keep taking the next step in the process.

Tip 38: Music is --- fifty/fifty

The truth is some people find music relaxing and helpful in their work. Others, however, find it too relaxing and they end up forgetting all about the task at hand.

You have to determine for yourself if music will serve as an aid to improving your focus or a distraction instead?

Tip 39: It is all about what you think and feel

Well-meaning friends may encourage you to try this and that to improve your focus. There is nothing wrong in listening to their advice. Remember, however, that every person is built differently. What may work for them may not work for you.

In the end, the best way to improve your focus is to do what works for *you* and not others.

Tip 40: Do not be a pushover

Some people will try to make you feel guilty about the time you are devoting to your goal. If your goal is important to you and not unethical or immoral, cruel, or harmful to yourself or anyone, then you have all the right in the world to devote yourself to it.

Tip 41: Do not allow emotional conflicts to get in your way

One of the worst kinds of distraction is emotional conflict. This kind of problem eats away at your concentration. If there is anything that is bothering you, resolve it right away before getting back to work.

Do not allow it to fester inside you. The longer you delay resolving such conflicts, the harder it will be to find a solution.

Tip 42: Know your priorities

If you are torn between doing two things, you have to give yourself an
ultimatum. Which is the more important priority – the goal you are working on or the alternative? Be brutally frank with yourself as you consider your options. If you have to choose then decide which of them are you willing to live without.

Tip 43: Consider your energy patterns

People have different energy patterns for various reasons. Some people, for instance, simply feel more energized to work in the middle of the night because there are fewer distractions.

Others like to work first thing in the morning because it makes them feel
productive. Their energy then wanes closer to lunch time but jumps back up when it is in the early evening.

Try to familiarize yourself with your energy pattern. Think back on the days you especially productive. When are you typically more efficient in completing your work? When are you less than diligent working on your tasks?

Tip 44: Maximize your time

Maximize your time by delegating appropriate tasks to other capable people. This allows you to concentrate on the most critical tasks.

Your focus will be fragmented if you have a million things to do and you are worrying the most about only a few of them. This is a recipe for mental paralysis.

Do yourself a favour. Find people whom you can trust to do a part of your work. Then devote yourself to doing what you feel needs the most of your attention.

Tip 45: Break things down into manageable pieces

Say you were given one whole cake to eat. Should you swallow it down in one bite? It would be pretty impossible to make an entire cake fit in your mouth, but you can definitely eat it all if you cut it into several slices. From there, you can eat a slice of cake one bite after another.

Sometimes, focusing on the bigger picture alone is not helpful. There are times when you have to forget about the bigger picture for a while and concentrate on one part of the picture at a time.

Tip 46: Make allowances for mistakes

Nobody is perfect. There will be times when nothing you can do is right. It is critical that you prepare beforehand for this and make allowances for mistakes.

If you can complete a task in thirty minutes, try giving yourself forty minutes instead. This way, you will not be terribly backed up if you make a mistake or two. Giving yourself allowances will also prevent your mistakes from breaking your stride. You will keep going – no matter what – like an Energizer bunny!

Tip 47: Practice memory improvement techniques

Memory and focus are intertwined in many ways. As such, improving your memory will consequently improve your ability to concentrate.

There are many ways to improve your concentration. You can find free exercises online or in the resources at the end of this book. You can also try joining a memory training workshop or read a memory enhancement book. There are also memory training software programs that you could try.

Tip 48: Learn how to read effectively

Whether your goal Is personal, work-related, or something else, there will be a time when your goal requires you to read something.

The world's fastest readers do not really read every. Rather, most speed readers are good at skimming and finding context clues. Their mind and eyes are trained to find the most important parts of each page and paragraph. Even if they have a limited amount of time to finish reading something, they will not have any problems grasping the most essential points of the text.

The written word is one of the most common things that many people have a hard time focusing on. You can avoid this problem if you just take the time to learn how to read effectively.

Tip 49: Be eager to learn

No one is too smart to stop learning. You will have an easier time focusing on new topics or tasks if train yourself *not* to be reluctant to learn about new things.

Granted, old dogs have a hard time learning new tricks, but surely you have more brain cells and willpower than canines?

Knowledge is a beautiful thing, and you should not turn your back on the
opportunity to learn something new if it will help you.

Tip 50: Remind yourself of the consequences

If you are tempted to give up on what you are doing, remind yourself of the consequences of not achieving your goal. If they are significant then you will get back on track.

Say you want to lose weight. If you eat that extra cup of rice tonight, it will mean having to spend an extra hour in the gym tomorrow. If you fail to do that, it will mean having your weight increase by two pounds. That, in turn, means not being able to fit into that new swimsuit you wanted to wear to the beach party – which the guy of your dreams is sure to attend.

Now ask yourself again – do you still want to give up on your goal and eat that cup of rice?

Tip 51: Remind yourself that you are not the only one at stake

Most of the time the goals you want to achieve affect others as well. Say it is your goal to increase profits by 25% by the end of the year. If you do not reach your goal in time, then you will not be able to give your staff the Christmas party and end-of-the-year bonuses they so richly deserve.

Tip 52: Forward all calls to your voice mail box

If you do not care about the consequences you will suffer by losing focus, then consider how those depending on you might be impacted.

Phones are also a source of distraction. Change your phone's message to let people know that you absolutely cannot afford to be disturbed.

Be sure, however, to let them know that you will be checking your email and voice message inbox regularly. Just because the phone rings does not mean you always have to answer right then.

<u>Tip 53: Limit you email-checking to five minutes per hour</u>

It doesn't need to be more than that because you should only reply to emails that are absolutely require a response. Anything less than important should be set aside. You have to be very firm about this rule or you will end up procrastinating on your goal again.

Tips to Get Motivated!

Tip 54: Remember that checklist? Do not forget to tick it off!

Seeing your checklist nearly completed will always work as a great boost to your confidence and motivation. If you were able to accomplish so much already, surely you can accomplish the rest of your tasks?

Tip 55: Use affirmations

Affirmations are basically positive statements that you tell to yourself repeatedly like a mantra. These are supposed to help you enjoy a positive frame of mind and be more confident about accomplishing your goal.

Some people say that affirmations should not use potential forms of verbs like "I can". In order to convince themselves of their abilities, affirmations should start with words such as "I will…" and "I am…" because you are *that* sure about yourself. Give it a try if you think it might work for you.

Tip 56: Think of *internal* rewards to congratulate yourself

Positive reinforcement is always a good thing so give yourself a pat on the back when you have completed an important or challenging step in your goal action plan.

Tip 57: Reward yourself materially as well.

Material rewards certainly matter. It does not have anything extravagant. If it is something you can afford and truly want, then you can also promise yourself a big reward when you reach your goal.

Try to be a little creative about your rewards. You can pamper yourself with a massage, take a trip out of town, or allow yourself a night out dining in the most expensive restaurant in town.

It can also be something as simple as letting yourself laze away over the
weekend, doing nothing and enjoying other small luxuries that you usually do not have time for.

Ultimately, just think about what will make you happy – and do it!

Tip 58: Reassess your goal

Sometimes the reason why you have a hard time motivating yourself is because your goal is no longer important. From time to time, you should re-evaluate your goal and find out if it still as important or it needs a little redefining.

Tip 59: Always search for the brighter side

Do not think that there is *no* brighter side because there always is. If you feel you have hit rock bottom, there is still a bright side. When you are down, there is no way else but *up!* I once heard a motivation teacher say, *"If you're face down in the ditch, at least turn over and see the sun!"*

Tip 60: Look for a role model

A role model does not have to be someone perfect, famous, or even older than you. Rather, a role model just has qualities that you so admire because you will become a better person for it.

When you feel like giving up, think about your role model. No one is immune to getting discouraged, but every person has the power to say 'no' to it. Your role model was strong enough to say 'no' to distraction and stay focused. Surely you can do it, too?

In the end, both of you are flesh and blood mortals – capable of doing the same thing as long as you put your mind to it.

Tip 61: Search for inspiration

Role models are different from inspiration. Role models are someone you try to emulate. People, things, or places that inspire you are also like goals. Why is becoming wealthy your goal? It is because you want to give your parents a chance to retire early. Then your parents are your inspiration.

If that were your goal, and you have become extremely frustrated so that you feel like throwing in the towel, picture your parents and what they will be like if they have to continue working for years in spite of their frail health. There is the inspiration to keep going.

Tip 62: Do not fail to take advantage of the power of visualization

It is easier to keep yourself motivated when you are able to visualize reaching your dream. Close your eyes and try to imagine what would happen if you were to reach your goal. How would it feel? What would happen afterwards? How would your life and others be impacted?

Make it so vivid that you can actually feel the joy of reaching your dream.

Tip 63: Proverbs are there for a reason

If you have noticed, proverbs and old sayings have been used throughout this book quite frequently. That is because they are true.

If there are no words you can think of personally to get yourself motivated, do not hesitate to call in the power of proverbs.

Tip 64: Talk to children

Kids say the darnedest things indeed, but they also often have an ingenuous way of seeing things. Their view of the world is untainted by cynicism and greed. Children can get you back to seeing the world with rose-coloured glasses.

Tip 65: *Carpe diem*

That is Latin for 'seize the day' if you have forgotten. Tell yourself that the opportunity your goal represents comes only once in a lifetime. If you do not seize the day – or the moment for that matter – then that chance may never come again.

Are you willing to take that risk?

Tip 66: Think of the last time you worked against all odds – and won

You are a powerful person yet sometimes you may need to remind yourself of that fact. If your confidence has taken a nosedive for any reason, think back to the last time you worked against all odds. Think of the time that no one had your back and only you had faith in yourself. Think of the time you had taken the role of an underdog – and won.

You did it then. You can do it again. Just believe!

Tip 67: Join motivation seminars now and then

If you have never tried attending a motivation seminar, it is easy for you to say that these so-called self-help gurus are just out to con you out of your money. Why not give it a try? At the most, you will only lose a couple of dollars for attending. Yet what if it works? Then you would have gained so much more!

The great motivational speaker Zig Ziglar once said (and I paraphrase) … *A motivation speech is like a bath, the effects of it where off after a while. However, it is a good idea to take another one.*

Tip 68: Remember the little things

Motivation is also a matter of perspective. If you are tired of working or doing something for the sake of achieving your goal alone, then do it just for the sake of doing it.

Do it because you are having fun doing it. Do it because you love it, and it makes you feel good. More often than not, the journey counts for more than the actual destination.

Tip 69: Keep a gratitude journal

For each day, try to think of as many things as you can that you are sincerely thankful for.

If you feel that you have absolutely nothing to be thankful about, then you are wrong. You are alive, aren't you? You can still read this and perhaps take up a pen and write your first post in your 'thank you' journal, can't you? That already gives you three reasons to be thankful about.

Remember: motivation is a matter of perspective. If you cannot see it from one angle, then you probably can from another.

Tip 70: Are you tempted to give up? Do (Insert Number Here) more

When you feel like you have reached the end of your tether, make one last big push by doing 5 more. Or if you are just one step away from giving in to exhaustion or sleep then do just 3 or even just one more!

You may not have completed your schedule for today but knowing that you gave it your best is enough to give you an energetic and motivated for the next day.

Tip 71: Failure is *not* an option

Granted, you are not stuck flying in Apollo 13. You just have to imagine yourself in the same back-against-the-wall scenario and that is sure to be motivation enough to work hard.

Tip 72: Never say never – unless it is to say you will *never* quit

You may change tactics, rest for a while, and redefine your goal but none of that means you are quitting. Never should *never* be a part of your

vocabulary – even if that sounds contradictory;
the moment you start entertaining doubts is the
moment you start losing.

Tip 73: Aim to be *better* and not perfect

Aiming to be perfect is setting yourself up for a lot
of disappointment and
discouragement. You will never be mistake free,
infallible, and perfect this side of Heaven. But
what you can do is to improve yourself and make
yourself or your situation better.

You may not be able to land on the moon, but if
you were to arm yourself with a telescope, then
the moon would be a lot closer.

Tip 74: Hope for the best but prepare for the worst

Motivation can be a double-edged sword. On one
hand, it can pierce the clouds of depression and
doubts. Especially when your motivation pays off
and you succeed in what you are trying to
achieve.

But what if you do not get what you want?
Motivation can end up hurting you. It seems like
you set yourself up for a fall. This *will* happen if
you have not prepared yourself for the potential
failure.

Preparing yourself for the worst just means that
you at least have considered the possibility – and
taken the necessary steps for dealing with it.

Tip 75: Do it – no matter how long it takes

It is very important that you do not give up on your goal just because your route to success turned out to be longer and more twisted than expected. At the end of the day the journey will mean more than getting to the destination.

Tip 76: Do not allow any source of frustration, problems, or depression to get worse. Eliminate it right away

If there is anything troubling you and making it difficult for you to stay focused and motivated – get rid of it right away. Nip it in the bud and do not wait for it to turn into a full-fledged disaster.

Tip Number 77: Think of all those who did not reach as far as you have come

If you were to crow out loud about your victories, then this would be boasting. But that is not what you are doing. You are just quietly reflecting on how far you have gone and what you have achieved that others cannot.

People have a tendency to keep on comparing themselves to others they feel are better. They fail to realize how much they have done more than the others.

When you realize that, you will see for yourself that accomplishing more than others does not make you better. You just happened to be more persistent, more patient, more methodical or maybe even lucky. The same goes for those who have done more than you.

Motivation is also a matter of time. You will get to your goal – you just have to work hard and keep your eyes on your destination.

Conclusion

At the end of the day, there is one final thought that you should remind yourself of when contemplating your next step:

The only difference between someone who succeeded and some who failed is that one of them *stopped trying.*

www.ingramcontent.com/pod-product-compliance
Lightning Source LLC
Chambersburg PA
CBHW072330270726
48658CB00016B/2241